DR. J. K. EVANS

THE TRUTH ABOUT CANCER

Learn How to Defeat Cancer and Live a Longer, Healthier Life.

Contents

Chapter 1: Introduction

What is cancer?

Cancer is a disease of the body's cells. Normally cells grow and multiply in a controlled way, however, sometimes cells become abnormal and keep growing. Abnormal cells can form a mass called a tumor.

Cancer is a term used to refer to the growth and potential spread of abnormal cells within the body. As cancerous cells can arise from almost any type of tissue cell, cancer refers to about 100 different diseases.

How does cancer develop and spread?

As mutant cells (those with mistakes in their genetic blueprint) grow and divide, a mass of abnormal cells, or a tumor, is formed. In some cases, these cells will form a discrete lump, in other cases such as leukemia, abnormal blood cells are in the body.

Cancer cells can break away from the mass (or tumor) and travel via the bloodstream or lymphatic system to different parts of the body. These cells can settle in other parts of the body to form a secondary cancer or metastasis.

Cancer can cause premature death because these secondary cancers stop parts of the body from working properly.

Types of cancer

Breast Cancer: Breast cancer can develop in both men and women but is more common in women. It commonly begins in the milk ducts or lobules of the breast tissue. Risk factors include age, family history, genetic mutations (e.g., BRCA1 and BRCA2), hormone therapy, and certain lifestyle variables.

Various treatments are available, such as surgical procedures, radiation treatment, chemotherapy, hormone therapy, and targeted therapy.

Lung Cancer: Lung cancer is typically separated into two basic types: non-small cell lung cancer (NSCLC) and small cell lung cancer (SCLC). Smoking is the leading cause of lung cancer, but exposure to environmental pollutants including asbestos and radon gas can dramatically raise the risk. Treatment relies on the sort and stage of lung cancer but may involve surgery, radiation therapy, chemotherapy, targeted therapy, or immunotherapy.

Prostate Cancer: Prostate cancer mainly affects elderly men and normally grows slowly. Risk factors include age, family history, and certain genetic variants. Treatment options range from active surveillance (monitoring without immediate treatment) to surgery, radiation therapy, hormone therapy, chemotherapy, or immunotherapy.

Colo rectal Cancer: This cancer can occur in the colon (large intestine) or rectum. Risk factors include age, family history, particular genetic disorders, and lifestyle factors such as food and physical exercise. Screening with colonoscopy can help detect precancerous polyps. Treatment involves surgery, radiation therapy, chemotherapy, targeted therapy, or immunotherapy.

Skin Cancer: The three main varieties of skin cancer are basal cell carcinoma, squamous cell carcinoma, and melanoma. Ultraviolet (UV) radiation from the sun and tanning beds is a considerable risk factor for skin cancer. Early diagnosis and removal are crucial. Treatment depends on the type and stage but may require surgery, radiation therapy, immunotherapy, or targeted therapy.

Ovarian Cancer: Ovarian cancer is frequently nicknamed the "silent killer" because it may not display evident indicators until it reaches an advanced stage. Risk factors include age, family history, certain genetic variations (e.g., BRCA1 and BRCA2), and characteristics related to reproductive history and hormone use. Treatment involves surgery, chemotherapy, targeted therapy, and, in some instances, radiation therapy.

Cervical Cancer: Most cervical cancers are caused by certain strains of HPV. Regular screening with Pap smears and HPV testing can reveal precancerous changes.

Various treatments are available, such as surgical procedures, radiation treatments, chemotherapy, and targeted therapies.

Pancreatic Cancer: Pancreatic cancer is often detected at an advanced stage, which makes it difficult to cure. Risk factors include smoking, family history, and certain genetic mutations. Treatment may consist of surgery, chemotherapy, radiation therapy, targeted therapy, or immunotherapy.

Risk factors for cancer

Cancer risk is most commonly used to denote the likelihood that a person will acquire cancer. In cancer care, this phrase is occasionally used to describe the possibility that the cancer may come back following therapy.

When cancer reappears, it is referred to as a recurrence.

Research studying cancer risk helps improve the health of many people. For example, when scientists established that smoking raises the risk of lung cancer, anti-smoking campaigns began and have helped save countless lives.

It is also crucial for people to identify their risk of having cancer. Knowing your specific risk factors can help you make decisions about your health and activities that can minimize your risk of having cancer and/or increase your likelihood of diagnosing cancer at an earlier stage. Cancer that is discovered in an early stage may be easier to treat or have a better prognosis.

1. Tobacco Use: Smoking is the single most avoidable cause of cancer worldwide. It is associated with several types of cancer, including lung, oral, throat, esophageal, bladder, and pancreatic cancer. Chewing tobacco and exposure to secondhand smoke are also significant risk factors.

2. Diet: A diet high in processed foods, red meat, and saturated fats, while deficient in fruits, vegetables, and fiber, is connected with an enhanced risk of cancer. This food habit can contribute to obesity and accelerate the development of cancer.

3. Obesity: Excess body weight, especially when centered around the belly, is an established risk factor for cancer. Obesity is connected to an increased risk of breast, colorectal, renal, pancreatic, and uterine malignancies, among others.

4. Physical Inactivity: A sedentary lifestyle without regular physical activity is connected with an elevated risk of cancer. Exercise helps regulate hormones, increase immune function, and lower inflammation, all of which can cut cancer risk.

5. UV Radiation: Exposure to ultraviolet (UV) radiation from the sun and tanning beds can lead to skin cancer, including melanoma, the worst type of skin cancer. Sunscreen and protective garments can help minimize this danger.

6. Environmental Carcinogens: Certain chemicals and compounds ubiquitous in the environment, such as asbestos, benzene, and radon gas, are established carcinogens and can boost the risk of cancer in people exposed to them.

7. Family History and Genetics: A family history of cancer can indicate a genetic predisposition to the disease. Some hereditary gene abnormalities, such as BRCA1 and BRCA2, greatly boost the risk of breast, ovarian, and other cancers.

8. Infections: Infections with specific viruses and bacteria can enhance cancer risk. For example, persistent HPV infections can lead to cervical and other cancers, while hepatitis B and C infections are connected to liver cancer.

9. Age: Cancer risk increases with age. Many types of cancer are more common in elderly persons because the cumulative effects of genetic defects and environmental exposures throughout time boost the likelihood of cancer formation.

10. Hormones: Exogenous hormones, such as those in hormone

replacement therapy (HRT) and certain birth control procedures, can increase cancer risk. For example, long-term usage of combination estrogen-progestin HRT has been connected with an elevated risk of breast cancer.

11. Radiation Exposure: High quantities of ionizing radiation exposure, whether through medical imaging procedures like CT scans or radiation therapy for other medical problems, can enhance the risk of cancer in exposed tissues.

12. Chronic Inflammation: Chronic inflammation is connected with an elevated risk of cancer. Conditions like inflammatory bowel disease (IBD) can lead to chronic inflammation in the gastrointestinal system, enhancing the risk of colorectal cancer.

13. Occupational Hazards: Certain jobs expose workers to carcinogens, such as asbestos for construction workers or benzene for chemical sector staff. Occupational exposure can greatly increase the incidence of different cancers.

leading to injury-related malignancies) or having unprotected intercourse with numerous partners (increasing the risk of HPV-related cancers) can contribute to cancer risk.

Understanding these risk factors is crucial for cancer prevention. Making excellent lifestyle choices, such as eliminating smoking, keeping a healthy weight, engaging in regular physical activity, and protecting oneself from environmental dangers and illnesses, can help lessen the risk of developing cancer. Regular screenings and early detection are also crucial for improving cancer outcomes. Individuals concerned about their cancer risk should speak with healthcare providers for specific information and screening ideas.

Symptoms of cancer

Very heavy night sweats or fever

Sweating at night or having a high temperature (fever) could be caused by illnesses or a side effect of some drugs. It's also usually experienced by women around the time of the menopause. But speak to your doctor if you have particularly heavy, drenching night sweats, or an unexplainable fever.

Fatigue

There are several reasons why you may feel more weary than usual, particularly if you're going through a stressful event, or having trouble sleeping. But if you're feeling fatigued all the time, or, for no clear reason, it could be an indication that something is wrong - speak to your doctor.

Unexplained bleeding or bruising

Unexplained bleeding or bruising when you have not hurt yourself is vital to have checked out by your doctor. This includes blood in your feces or pee, as well as vomiting or coughing up blood. It also covers any unexplainable vaginal bleeding between periods, after intercourse or after the menopause. No matter how much blood or what color it is (blood can be red, or a deeper tint like brown or black), speak to your doctor.

Unexplained discomfort or ache

Pain is one way our body warns us that something is amiss. As we age older, it's more natural to have aches and pains. But unexplainable or persistent pain elsewhere in the body could be an indication of something more harmful.

Unexplained weight loss

Small weight fluctuations over time are normally common, but if you have lost a large amount of weight without trying to, inform your doctor.

Unusual bulges or expansion everywhere

Persistent lumps or swelling in any part of your body should be dealt with seriously. This includes any bumps in the neck, armpit, stomach, groin, chest, breast, or testicle.

Diagnosis of cancer

Medical History and Physical Examination:

During the medical history interview, the healthcare provider will ask about the patient's personal medical history, including any past illnesses, surgeries, prescriptions, and lifestyle variables such as smoking or exposure to environmental toxins.

Family history is particularly crucial, as many malignancies can have a hereditary component. Knowing if close relatives have had cancer can assist in determining the patient's risk.

Imaging Tests:

X-rays are widely used to diagnose bone abnormalities and, in certain cases, lung malignancies. They include exposing the body to a small amount of radiation.

Computed Tomography (CT) scans produce detailed cross-sectional images of the body, allowing for the identification of tumors and anomalies in numerous organs.

Magnetic Resonance Imaging (MRI) employs powerful magnets and radio waves to make detailed images of soft tissues like the brain, spinal cord, and muscles.

Ultrasound employs high-frequency sound waves to create images of organs, helping diagnose illnesses including breast, thyroid, or pelvic malignancies.

Positron Emission Tomography (PET) scans are widely used to measure metabolic activity in the body and can assist in locating malignant tumors.

Blood Tests:

Blood tests can evaluate certain markers or compounds in the blood that may be related to cancer. For instance, elevated levels of prostate-specific antigen (PSA) can indicate prostate cancer and elevated CA-125 values can signify ovarian cancer.

Complete blood counts (CBC) can detect abnormalities in blood cell counts, which may be a symptom of blood malignancies such as leukemia or lymphoma.

Biopsy:

Biopsies are the gold standard for verifying cancer diagnoses. They entail taking a sample of tissue or cells from a questionable location.

Needle biopsies are routinely done for breast, lung, and prostate malignancies, among others. The sample is frequently guided by imaging tools like ultrasound or CT scans.

Surgical biopsies may be essential when a larger tissue sample is desired or when the tumor is readily accessible.

Endoscopic biopsies are performed using a flexible tube with a camera (endoscope) and are typically utilized for gastrointestinal malignancies.

Histopathology and Laboratory Analysis:

The tissue or cell samples recovered from a biopsy are analyzed by a pathologist. The pathologist examines the look of the cells under a microscope to determine if they are malignant and identifies the type of cancer.

Tumor grade shows how aggressive the cancer cells appear, while staging determines the extent of the disease within the body.

Staging:

Staging is a vital step in cancer diagnosis and therapy planning. It helps assess the size of the tumor, whether it has migrated to adjacent lymph nodes, and whether it has metastasized (spread) to other organs.

Staging techniques like the TNM (Tumor, Nodes, Metastasis) scheme are routinely used to classify cancer stages.

Genetic Testing:

Genetic testing can discover particular mutations or abnormalities in a person's DNA that may raise their chance of acquiring certain types of cancer. For example, BRCA1 and BRCA2 mutations are associated with an increased risk of breast and ovarian malignancies.

Consultation with Specialists:

Once the diagnosis and staging are complete, patients are generally directed to a team of experts, including medical oncologists, surgical oncologists, radiation oncologists, and other healthcare professionals. Together, they construct a treatment plan suited to the patient's diagnosis and needs.

The diagnosis of cancer is a complex and precise process that requires the collaboration of numerous medical professionals. Early identification and correct diagnosis are critical for determining the most effective treatment options and boosting the odds of successful outcomes for people with cancer. Patients should actively interact with their healthcare team and seek a second opinion if necessary to obtain the best possible care.

Chapter 2: Cancer treatment options

Surgery:
Surgery is a frequent treatment for many forms of cancer, especially solid tumors. It involves the removal of cancerous tissue and is often the primary treatment for localized cancers.

Depending on the cancer's location and stage, surgery may involve removing a section of an organ (e.g., lumpectomy for breast cancer), the entire organ (e.g., prostatectomy for prostate cancer), or nearby lymph nodes.

Advances in surgical treatments, such as minimally invasive surgery and robotic-assisted surgery, have cut recuperation periods and post-operative issues.

Radiation Therapy:
Radiation therapy uses high-energy X-rays or other kinds of radiation to target and damage cancer cells. It can be used as a major treatment or in conjunction with surgery or chemotherapy.

External beam radiation therapy directs radiation from outside the body, while brachytherapy involves injecting radioactive sources directly into or around the tumor.

Radiation therapy is highly helpful in treating confined cancers, such as early-stage breast cancer, cervical cancer, and prostate cancer.

Chemotherapy:

Chemotherapy is the use of drugs that circulate throughout the body to kill rapidly dividing cells, particularly cancer cells.

It is commonly used in the treatment of several cancers, both as a principal treatment and in conjunction with other drugs.

Chemotherapy is administered in several ways, including intravenous (IV), oral, or injectable.

While useful, chemotherapy can generate unpleasant symptoms such as nausea, tiredness, and hair loss.

Targeted Therapy:

Targeted treatment drugs are designed to interfere with specific molecules or pathways involved in cancer growth and progression.

Unlike chemotherapy, which targets rapidly dividing cells throughout the body, targeted therapies are more precise and often have fewer side effects.

Examples of targeted therapies include tyrosine kinase inhibitors (TKIs) and monoclonal antibodies.

Immunotherapy:

Immunotherapy harnesses the body's immune system to discover and attack cancer cells.

Checkpoint inhibitors, such as pembrolizumab and nivolumab, target immunological checkpoints that hinder T cells from attacking cancer cells.

CAR-T cell treatment comprises genetically modifying a patient's T cells to target specific cancer antigens.

Immunotherapy has shown outstanding success in treating a range of malignancies, including melanoma, lung cancer, and certain kinds of lymphoma.

Hormone Therapy:

Hormone treatment is often used to treat hormone-sensitive cancers, such as breast and prostate cancer.

It functions by either decreasing the body's production of hormones or interfering with hormone receptors in cancer cells.

For example, tamoxifen is regularly given in breast cancer to block estrogen receptors.

Stem Cell Transplantation:

Stem cell transplantation is applied in the treatment of various blood cancers, like leukemia, lymphoma, and multiple myeloma.

It comprises restoring damaged or diseased bone marrow with healthy stem cells.

Autologous transplants employ the patient's stem cells, while allogeneic transplants use donor stem cells.

Precision Medicine:

Precision medicine, often known as personalized medicine, involves altering cancer treatment based on the precise genetic and molecular characteristics of the tumor.

Genetic testing helps reveal mutations and alterations that may react to targeted treatments or clinical trials.

Palliative Care:

Palliative care is a specific kind of medical care concentrating on enhancing the quality of life for persons with advanced or terminal cancer.

It focuses on pain management, symptom reduction, emotional support, and psychological well-being.

Clinical Trials:

Clinical trials are research studies that test new cancer treatments, medications, or therapies.

Participating in clinical trials can offer patients access to innovative medicines that may not be available through standard pharmaceuticals.

Cancer treatment regimens are extremely personalized and are established by collaboration among a patient's healthcare team, which may include medical oncologists, surgical oncologists, radiation oncologists, nurses, and other specialists. The choice of treatment depends on parameters such as the cancer sort, stage, genetic factors, overall health, and patient preferences. Patients need to have open and educated discussions with their healthcare specialists to make the best treatment decisions for their specific circumstances.

Chapter 3: New and emerging cancer treatments

Immunotherapy Combinations:

Immunotherapy has revolutionized cancer treatment by increasing the body's immune system to target and destroy cancer cells. Combining numerous immunotherapy medicines, such as checkpoint inhibitors like pembrolizumab and nivolumab, can boost response rates by targeting several immune evasion mechanisms.

Cancer Vaccines:

Cancer vaccines try to stimulate the immune system's response against cancer cells.

Therapeutic cancer vaccines, like Sipuleucel-T for prostate cancer, are designed to teach the immune system to recognize specific tumor antigens, perhaps leading to more effective and persistent immune responses.

Precision Oncology:

Precision medicine emphasizes tailoring treatment based on the genetic and molecular characteristics of a patient's cancer.

Targeted medicines, guided by genetic analysis, can target specific molecules or processes that promote cancer growth, resulting in more precise and effective treatment.

Liquid Biopsies:

Liquid biopsies require testing a patient's blood for circulating tumor DNA (ctDNA) or other markers.

These tests offer a non-invasive way to monitor cancer progression, detect minimum residual disease, and identify growing resistance mutations, enabling early therapeutic changes.

Nanotechnology:

Nanoparticles, typically composed of biocompatible materials, can transport drugs directly to cancer cells, raising drug concentration at the tumor location while minimizing systemic toxicity.

This approach can improve the efficacy of chemotherapy, radiation treatment, and targeted medicines.

CRISPR-Based Therapies:

CRISPR-Cas9 gene editing method permits for exact alteration of the DNA within cancer cells.

It holds the potential for rectifying cancer-promoting mutations and improving the immune system's ability to battle cancer.

Epigenetic Therapies:

Epigenetic changes influence gene expression. Drugs like azacitidine and decitabine reverse abnormal DNA methylation in blood cancers.

These drugs help restore normal gene function and limit cancer progression.

Hyperthermia:

Hyperthermia involves heating cancer tissues, making them more sensitive to radiation therapy or chemotherapy.

By improving blood flow to tumors, heat enhances therapy effectiveness and can be especially useful in restricted tumors.

These new cancer medicines bring hope for more effective and tailored therapies, decreased side effects, and improved patient outcomes. However, it's vital to understand that not all of these medicines are accessible for routine clinical usage, and many are still in the research and development phase or limited to specific illness categories. Patients exploring these therapies should connect with their healthcare specialists and consider joining in clinical trials when suitable to acquire the newest discoveries in cancer care.

Chapter 4: Cancer prevention

Tobacco and Smoking Cessation:

Tobacco usage is the single most avoidable cause of cancer worldwide. It includes carcinogens (cancer-causing substances) that can damage DNA and lead to the formation of malignant cells.

Smoking stopping is one of the most effective treatments to minimize cancer risk. When a person quits smoking, the body begins to mend itself, and the risk of cancer lowers over time.

Limit Alcohol Consumption:

Excessive alcohol usage is connected with an increased risk of numerous types of cancer, including mouth, throat, esophageal, liver, and breast cancer.

Reducing alcohol intake or abstinence can lessen cancer risk. It's suggested that ladies have no more than one alcoholic drink per day, while males should limit alcohol to no more than two drinks per day.

Maintain a Healthy Diet:

Maintaining a nutritious diet is essential for reducing the risk of cancer. Foods rich in fruits, vegetables, healthy grains, and lean meats supply important nutrients and antioxidants that help protect cells from damage.

Limiting processed foods, sugary snacks, and red meat can minimize the intake of chemicals that are connected to cancer risk.

Physical Activity:

Regular physical activity not only helps maintain a healthy weight but also has direct benefits in cancer prevention. Exercise can reduce the incidence of colon, breast, and endometrial cancers.

It is recommended to engage in at least 150 minutes of moderate-intensity physical activity or 75 minutes of vigorous-intensity exercise each week.

Weight Management:

Obesity is connected with an increased risk of several malignancies, including breast, colorectal, kidney, and endometrial cancer.

Achieving and maintaining a healthy weight with a balanced diet and frequent physical activity helps lessen cancer risk.

Sun Protection:

Overexposure to ultraviolet (UV) radiation from the sun is a known risk factor for skin cancer, notably melanoma, the most lethal type of skin cancer.

Sun protection strategies, such as wearing sunscreen, protective garments, and eye wear, can minimize the risk of UV-induced skin damage.

Vaccinations:

Vaccines can prevent certain cancer-causing disorders. The HPV vaccine protects against human papillomavirus, which can lead to cervical, anal, and oropharyngeal cancers.

The hepatitis B vaccine reduces the incidence of liver cancer, as chronic hepatitis B infection is a primary risk factor.

Screening and Early Detection:
Regular cancer screenings can find cancer at an early, more treatable stage. Mammograms, colonoscopies, Pap smears, and other screenings are crucial for early detection and prevention.
Follow specified screening criteria based on your age, gender, and family history.

Avoid Environmental Carcinogens:
Limit exposure to recognized carcinogens, such as asbestos, radon gas, and occupational chemicals. Follow safety requirements and implement protective measures as applicable.

Genetic Counseling and Testing:
If you have a family history of cancer or known genetic defects related to cancer risk (e.g., BRCA1 and BRCA2), consider genetic counseling and testing to assess your risk and make informed decisions for cancer prevention.

Reduce Stress:
Chronic stress may impair the immune system and may raise cancer risk. Engage in stress-reduction practices such as meditation, yoga, or mindfulness to promote general well-being.

Limit Hormone Replacement Therapy (HRT):
Long-term administration of hormone replacement medication, especially estrogen and progesterone, may increase the risk of various malignancies, such as breast cancer.
If HRT is necessary for menopausal symptoms, discuss the risks and benefits with your healthcare practitioner and research non-hormonal

alternatives.

Breastfeed if Possible:
Breastfeeding has been related to a decreased risk of breast and ovarian cancer in mothers.

Whenever possible, breastfeeding can offer both maternal and newborn health benefits.

Regular Health Check-ups:
Routine medical check-ups can assist in revealing risk factors and conditions that may increase cancer risk. Regular visits to healthcare providers can lead to early intervention and prevention activities.

Implementing these cancer prevention strategies can drastically lessen the risk of contracting cancer and enhance general health. It's vital to adopt a holistic approach to prevention by integrating numerous strategies and having a healthy lifestyle. Consulting with healthcare specialists for tailored guidance based on individual risk factors is highly crucial in cancer prevention.

Chapter 5: Living with cancer

Coping with a cancer diagnosis

Coping with a cancer diagnosis is an emotional and demanding process that involves several ways to help individuals and their loved ones negotiate the medical, emotional, and practical elements of cancer. Here's a more extensive explanation of the important stages of coping with a cancer diagnosis:

Seek Emotional Support:

Receiving a cancer diagnosis can provoke a wide range of feelings, including fear, worry, anger, and grief. It's crucial to discuss these feelings with trusted friends and family members who can offer understanding and empathy.

Consider attending a cancer support group or getting individual counseling or therapy to connect with people who are going through similar situations and obtain professional help.

Educate Yourself:

Learning about your cancer diagnosis, its stage, treatment options, and potential side effects can empower you to make informed decisions regarding your healthcare.

Seek information from trusted sources such as your healthcare team, respected cancer organizations, and medical literature. Avoid relying only on internet searches, as not all sources are accurate or up-to-date.

Build a Strong Support System:

Lean on your network of family and friends for emotional support. Let them know your specific demands and boundaries so that they can provide efficient support.

Designate a caregiver or advocate who can accompany you to medical appointments, take notes, and assist with practical duties.

Communicate with Your Healthcare Team:

Establish clear and open communication with your medical team, including oncologists, nurses, and other healthcare experts. Ask questions, convey your concerns, and seek clarification regarding your treatment plan.

Don't hesitate to obtain a second opinion if you have reservations about your diagnosis or treatment alternatives.

Maintain a Healthy Lifestyle:

A proper diet is vital during cancer treatment. Consult with a licensed dietician who specializes in cancer care to design a balanced diet that supports your overall health and well-being.

Engage in physical activity as tolerated, as it can help reduce fatigue, boost mood, and enhance your quality of life.

Manage Stress:

Cancer diagnosis and treatment can be distressing. Explore stress-reduction strategies such as meditation, mindfulness, deep breathing exercises, or yoga to increase emotional and psychological well-being.

Consider seeking professional support from a therapist or counselor who specializes in cancer-related issues to handle the emotional obstacles that may occur.

Set Realistic Goals and Priorities:

Understand that your daily routine and priorities may alter throughout cancer treatment. Focus on self-care and managing treatment-related adverse effects.

Set reasonable short-term goals to sustain a sense of accomplishment and development.

Explore Complementary Therapies:

Some patients find relief from cancer-related symptoms and stress through alternative therapies including acupuncture, massage, or relaxation techniques. Discuss these choices with your healthcare team to confirm they are safe and acceptable for your condition.

Maintain a Journal:

Keeping a journal can be therapeutic, allowing you to express your thoughts and emotions, track symptoms, and capture questions for your healthcare staff.

It can also act as a record of your journey, emphasizing your progress and resilience.

Accept Help and Support:

Be open to accepting help from friends and relatives who sincerely wish to assist you. People typically appreciate specific requests for support, such as transportation to appointments or help with household duties.

Allowing people to provide emotional and practical support might reduce some of the challenges you may experience.

Plan for the Future:

Address legal and financial problems, including wills, advance directives, and financial planning, with the support of a lawyer or financial counselor.

Having these preparations in place can bring peace of mind and guarantee your preferences are honored.

Stay Positive but Realistic:

While having an optimistic view might be advantageous, it's necessary to recognize and address negative feelings as well. It's natural to experience fear, anger, sadness, or irritation.

Focus on the current moment and enjoy tiny triumphs and milestones along the way.

Celebrate Life:

Continue to engage in activities you enjoy and spend quality time with loved ones. Celebrate key occasions and milestones, especially during treatment.

Maintaining a sense of routine and finding moments of delight can boost your spirits and enhance your overall well-being.

Coping with a cancer diagnosis is a deeply personal journey, and everyone's experience is unique.

It is essential to be tolerant of oneself and to seek expert assistance when necessary. Your healthcare staff can provide information on managing symptoms and side effects, as well as connect you with options for emotional and psychological support. With the correct support, a proactive attitude to self-care, and a resilient mindset, many individuals successfully manage their cancer journey and find strength in the face of hardship.

Managing side effects of cancer treatment:

Managing the side effects of cancer treatment is an important feature of the cancer journey. Cancer medicines like chemotherapy, radiation therapy, immunotherapy, and targeted therapy can often lead to severe side effects that can be physically and emotionally exhausting. Effective control of these side effects is crucial to enhance your overall quality of life throughout treatment. Here's a more detailed explanation of strategies for managing normal cancer medication side effects:

Nausea and Vomiting:

Cancer treatment can often cause nausea and vomiting as a side effect. Your healthcare provider can offer antiemetic medications to avoid or control these symptoms.

Adjust your diet by eating small, frequent meals and choosing bland, easy-to-digest foods.

Natural remedies like ginger, acupuncture, or relaxation techniques may bring comfort to certain individuals.

Fatigue:

Cancer-related fatigue can be scary. Balance your workout intensity with rest, and listen to your body's suggestions.

Prioritize tasks and allocate duties to conserve your energy.

A well-balanced diet and staying hydrated can help combat tiredness.

Hair Loss:

Hair loss, particularly with chemotherapy, can be emotionally difficult. Consider cutting your hair short before treatment to make hair loss less visible.

Use modest hair care products and avoid severe treatments.

Wearing wigs, scarves, or hats could assist in increasing your self-esteem throughout hair loss.

Mouth Sores and Taste Changes:

Mouth sores can be controlled by maintaining good oral hygiene, including using a soft toothbrush and alcohol-free mouthwash.

Avoid spicy, acidic, or hot foods that can irritate your mouth.

Stay hydrated, and try with cold or room-temperature foods if your taste is disrupted.

Diarrhea and Constipation:

Hydration is crucial when managing diarrhea to prevent dehydration.

It is important to stay hydrated. Make sure to consume adequate amounts of fluids.

A high-fiber diet can help prevent constipation, but avoid high-fiber meals during periods of diarrhea.

Medications offered by your healthcare team can help treat both diarrhea and constipation.

Neutropenia (Low White Blood Cell Count):

Neutropenia raises the probability of infection. Practice tight cleanliness, including frequent handwashing, and avoid crowds and sick individuals.

Your healthcare provider may offer medications like growth factors to increase white blood cell production.

Anemia (Low Red Blood Cell Count):

Anemia can contribute to fatigue and weakness. Iron supplements or medicines may be supplied.

Consume a diet rich in iron, such as lean meats, beans, and leafy green vegetables.

Rest and participate in light activities to conserve energy.

Skin Changes:

Dryness, itching, and sensitivity are prevalent skin issues following cancer therapy. Use gentle, fragrance-free skin care products.

Protect your skin from the sun and harsh temperatures.

Inform your healthcare practitioner about any skin changes, as they may advise specialized lotions or ointments.

Peripheral Neuropathy:

It is important to inform your healthcare team if you experience numbness, tingling, or weakness in your hands and feet, as these can be signs of peripheral neuropathy.

Prioritize safety to prevent falls or injuries. Use handrails, wear non-slip shoes, and avoid hot showers.

Physical therapy or medicines may help control neuropathy symptoms.

Emotional and Psychological Support:

Reach out to those close to you for emotional support, or consider speaking with a counselor. Numerous cancer treatment centers provide counseling services. To help manage stress and anxiety, try relaxation methods, mindfulness, or meditation.

Consider attending a support group to connect with people facing similar concerns.

Pain:

Report any pain to your healthcare team promptly.

They can modify your pain management strategy as necessary.

Non-pharmacological therapy such as heat or cold packs, massage, and acupuncture may help ease pain.

Lymphedema:

If you experience swelling, especially after lymph node surgery, visit a lymphedema specialist for evaluation and management.

Compression gear and particular workouts can help decrease lymphedema.

Cognitive Changes ("Chemo Brain"):

Cognitive abnormalities including memory difficulties could arise during cancer therapy. Keep a notebook, use calendars, and make lists to aid with organization.

Engage in mental activity and stay intellectually busy to help sustain cognitive function.

Sexual Health:

Cancer treatment can influence sexual function and desire. Open communication with your partner and healthcare personnel is crucial.

Seek guidance from a sexual health specialist or counselor if needed. Solutions like lubricants, hormone therapy, or physical therapy may be prescribed.

Financial and Practical Support:

Cancer therapy can be pricey. Explore financial support programs, insurance alternatives, and resources supplied by cancer groups.

Delegate responsibility or seek help with practical matters to decrease stress.

Managing cancer treatment side effects is a collaborative effort between you and your healthcare team. Open and honest communication is crucial to ensure your side effects are addressed effectively. Your healthcare team can give tailored guidance and interventions to suit your specific requirements and lessen the impact of side effects on your everyday life and well-being. Remember that obtaining aid and support from both medical specialists and your support network is a vital component of managing the challenges of cancer treatment.

Support resources for cancer patients and their families:

Support tools for cancer patients and their families are vital to assist individuals in coping with the physical, emotional, and practical issues that typically accompany a cancer diagnosis. Here's a more extensive overview of these assistance resources:

Cancer Centers and Hospitals:

These institutes are at the forefront of cancer care, offering a wide spectrum of medical knowledge and treatment choices.

In addition to medical care, cancer clinics often provide comprehensive support services, such as access to oncology social workers who can help patients and families negotiate the emotional and logistical obstacles of cancer.

Support Groups:

Cancer support groups play a critical role in delivering emotional support. They create a sense of belonging and understanding, allowing participants to communicate their concerns, hopes, and uncertainties in a secure and non-judgmental setting.

Support group members often discuss coping methods and practical advice for managing side effects and treatment-related issues.

National Cancer Organizations:

National cancer organizations like the American Cancer Society serve as reliable sources of information, advocacy, and support.

They spread vital resources, including booklets, online guides, and instructional materials that empower patients and their families to make informed decisions about their cancer journey.

Local Cancer Organizations:

Local cancer organizations are closely tied to their communities and provide individual help.

They may offer transportation services to help patients get to and from therapy, financial aid for medical expenditures, and support groups that meet in person.

Cancer Hotlines:

Hotlines are conveniently available resources that give instant assistance. They are manned by specialists who can address issues, provide emotional support, and guide callers to suitable services.

These hotlines can be particularly helpful during situations of crisis or when patients and families need immediate answers.

Psychosocial Support:

Cancer can take a severe emotional toll. Psychosocial support services help individuals cope with anxiety, sadness, and stress.

Social workers and mental health professionals cooperate with patients and families to develop coping techniques, manage loss, and enhance mental well-being.

Financial Assistance Programs:

The tremendous cost of cancer treatment can be a major challenge. These programs give financial support by helping cover the price of medical treatment, drugs, and other connected expenses.

Financial counselors can provide help with navigating insurance, negotiating medical bills, and accessing relevant resources.

Home Health Care Services:

Home healthcare professionals deliver medical competence and comfort to patients in their own homes. They can dispense prescriptions, manage symptoms, and provide important companionship.

These programs allow patients to receive treatment in a familiar and supportive environment.

Hospice and Palliative Care:

Hospice and palliative care teams focus on increasing the quality of life for patients with advanced cancer. They give pain and symptom treatment while addressing emotional and spiritual requirements.

Their services extend to aiding families during the end-of-life journey, offering assistance on loss and bereavement.

Nutritional Support:

A proper diet is vital during cancer treatment. Registered dietitians with expertise in oncology can establish tailored food programs to alleviate treatment-related side effects and maintain general health.

Nutritional support helps patients maintain strength and energy levels, which might be crucial during treatment.

Transportation Assistance:

Transportation services meet a practical need by ensuring that patients can go to medical appointments, even if they lack reliable transportation.

This support helps patients retain continuity of care and minimizes barriers to getting therapy.

Child and Adolescent Support:

Pediatric and adolescent cancer care groups provide specialized care for young patients and their families.

These organizations promote child-friendly surroundings, offer age-appropriate materials, and provide emotional support to children and their carers.

Online Communities and Forums:

Online groups and forums broaden the reach of support, uniting individuals worldwide who are afflicted by cancer.

These virtual places give a sense of community, information sharing, and emotional support 24/7, making them accessible and handy.

Legal and Advocacy Resources:

Legal assistance organizations and patient advocacy groups function as advocates for patients and their rights.

They offer advice on legal concerns, ensuring that patients are treated fairly and have access to required resources and rights.

Educational Workshops & Webinars:

Educational events give a forum for patients and families to learn about cancer-related issues, treatment alternatives, and self-care practices.

Attending these programs can enable individuals to take an active role in their care and make educated decisions.

Effective utilization of these support tools can dramatically improve the cancer experience for patients and their families, helping them negotiate the obstacles of diagnosis, treatment, and recovery with greater confidence and resilience. It's crucial to speak with healthcare providers and reach out to support organizations that correspond with your individual needs and concerns during your cancer experience. Additionally, soliciting the support of friends and family members can provide a strong network of emotional support and aid.

CONCLUSION

CONCLUSION

T HE TRUTH ABOUT CANCER" Your decision to explore this significant topic demonstrates your unwavering commitment to understanding and conquering one of the most challenging issues that humanity is currently facing. In the fight against cancer, I hope this book has given you insightful information, wisdom, and encouragement.

We have examined the intricacies of cancer, its causes, risk factors, prevention tactics, and the most recent developments in treatment choices across the chapters. We've examined how this disease has many facets and how sufferers and their loved ones can benefit from lifestyle adjustments, early identification, and cutting-edge medical advancements.

I want to express my gratitude to all the people and families who have been impacted by cancer. Your fortitude, resiliency, and resolve in the face of difficulty continue to motivate us all. I sincerely hope the material in this book serves as a ray of hope and equips you with the knowledge needed to make wise choices regarding cancer support, prevention, and treatment.

As we come to the end of our trip, I humbly beg for your assistance in spreading the word about "THE TRUTH ABOUT CANCER." Please think about writing a good review if you found this book to be educational, insightful, or even just thought-provoking. Your evaluations not only assist other readers in finding this beneficial resource, but they also give me insightful feedback that helps me enhance and improve subsequent editions.

Together, we can keep promoting cancer awareness, advancing research, and fighting for improved cancer treatment. Let's band together in the fight against cancer and work toward a time when finding a cure is more than just a pipe dream. May you live long, happy, and hopeful lives in gratitude for your trust and commitment.

With sincere appreciation,

(DR. J. K. EVANS)